MEDITERRANEAN DIET COOKBOOK

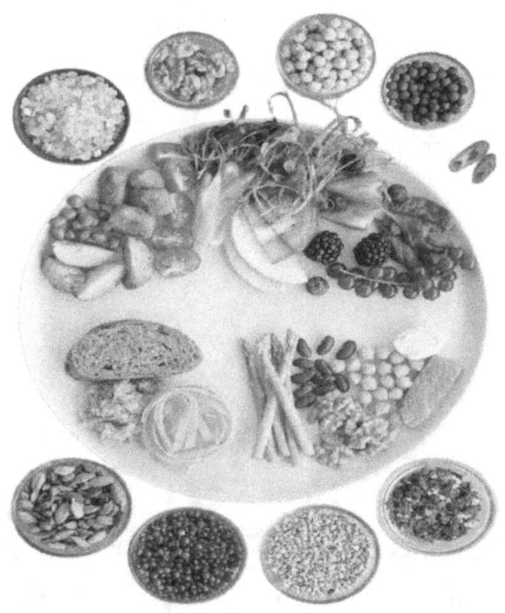

Delicious and Nutritious Recipes for a Healthier Mediterranean Diet

DR. KIMBERLY THORPE

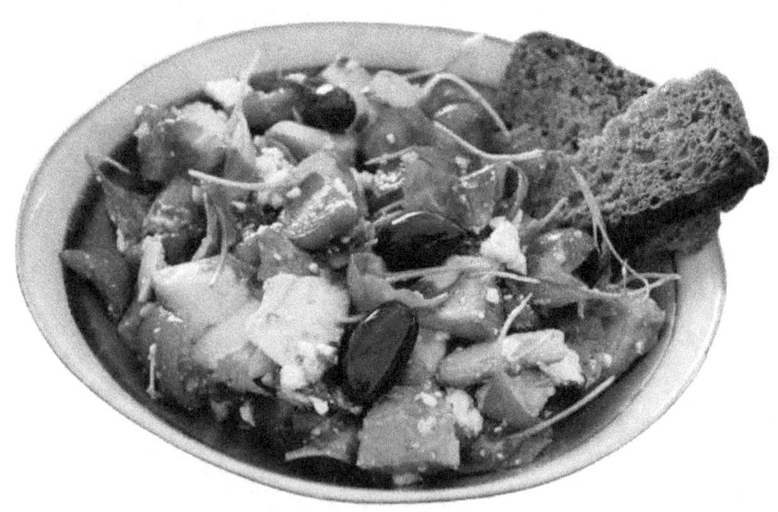

TABLE OF CONTENTS

CHAPTER THREE 47

MEDITERRANEAN GRAIN, PASTA AND RICE RECIPES

CHAPTER SIX 99

CHAPTER NINE 145

INTRODUCTION

Cynthia had been struggling to lose weight for over a year and was feeling discouraged. She had tried every diet imaginable, but none of them seemed to work for her. She was ready to give up when her friend suggested trying a Mediterranean diet.

Cynthia was a bit skeptical at first, but she decided to give it a try. She began by replacing processed foods with fresh, whole foods like fruits, vegetables, whole grains, legumes, and nuts. She also made sure to include healthy fats like olive oil and fish in her diet.

At first, Cynthia was a bit intimidated by the idea of eating this new way, but she quickly found that it was easier than she thought. She also found that the food was delicious and satisfying. The recipes were easy to make and didn't require a lot of time or effort.

After a few weeks, Cynthia began to notice a difference. She felt more energetic and her clothes were starting to fit better.

She was also losing weight. She was so encouraged that she kept up with the diet and continued to see results.

Cynthia was thrilled by the results of the Mediterranean diet. She was losing weight and feeling better than ever. She was so happy that she decided to stick with it and continue to enjoy all the delicious, healthy foods.

One of the most well-liked and healthiest diets in the world is the Mediterranean diet. It is based on the traditional cuisine of countries bordering the Mediterranean Sea, including Greece, Italy, Spain, and Morocco. This diet is known for its emphasis on fresh fruits and vegetables, legumes, whole grains, fish, olive oil, and nuts, as well as its moderate consumption of red wine and dairy products. The Mediterranean Diet is not only a delicious and nutritious way to eat, but also a lifestyle that encourages physical activity and a balanced lifestyle.

Focusing mostly on plant-based foods including fruits, vegetables, legumes, whole grains, nuts, and olive oil defines this diet. Meat, poultry, and dairy products are eaten in moderation, and fish is a major component of the diet. Red wine is also consumed in moderation as part of the Mediterranean Diet.

The Mediterranean Diet is not only delicious and nutritious, but it is also associated with a number of health benefits. Studies have shown that the Mediterranean Diet can help reduce the risk of heart disease, stroke, and type 2 diabetes, as well as help with weight loss. It has also been linked to a reduced risk of certain types of cancer and age-related cognitive decline.

Overall, the Mediterranean Diet is an excellent choice for anyone looking to improve their health and well-being. With its focus on fresh, healthy ingredients, this diet is easy to incorporate into your daily life. With its emphasis on physical activity, balanced lifestyle, and moderate consumption of red wine, the Mediterranean Diet may be the perfect choice for you!

Welcome to the world of Mediterranean cooking! In this cookbook, you will find an array of delicious, healthy recipes inspired by the traditional cuisines of countries such as Italy, Greece, Spain, and Morocco. All of the recipes are based on the Mediterranean diet, which is one of the healthiest eating patterns in the world.

The Mediterranean diet is focused on eating nutritious, unprocessed, and seasonal ingredients; emphasizing plant-based foods such as fruits, vegetables, whole grains, nuts, and legumes; and including moderate amounts of fish, poultry, and dairy. In addition to being incredibly healthy, the Mediterranean diet is also incredibly delicious. Get ready for a culinary journey through the Mediterranean! With these recipes, you will learn how to make flavorful dishes that are full of nutrition. Enjoy!

CHAPTER ONE

WHAT IS THE MEDITERRANEAN DIET?

The Mediterranean diet is a way of eating based on the traditional dietary habits of southern Italy, Crete, and other areas around the Mediterranean Sea. It is a diet that is largely plant-based, with an emphasis on whole grains, fruits, vegetables, nuts, and seeds. It also includes limited amounts of animal products such as poultry, eggs, fish, and dairy. Fat sources are mostly from olive oil and other plant-based sources, while added sugars and processed foods are generally avoided.

This style of eating has been associated with numerous health benefits, such as lower risks of heart disease, stroke, some cancers, and type 2 diabetes. Studies have also linked it to improved mental health, better weight management, and a longer life. It is regarded as one of the world's healthiest diets.

The Mediterranean Diet is based on the traditional foods that people used to eat in countries like Greece, Italy, and Spain before the introduction of highly processed foods. It is based on the idea that meals should be prepared from fresh, seasonal ingredients with plenty of fresh fruits, vegetables, whole grains, legumes, nuts, and seeds. It also includes healthy fats from olive oil and other plant-based sources, as well as fish and seafood. Red meat and processed foods should be avoided.

The Mediterranean Diet isn't a strict set of rules, but rather a way of eating that encourages mindful, healthy meal choices. It also encourages social gatherings with family and friends, who come together to break bread and enjoy the pleasure of eating.

Overall, the Mediterranean Diet is a balanced, healthy way of eating that is associated with numerous health benefits. It is also a great way to enjoy delicious meals and socialize with friends and family.

BENEFITS OF THE MEDITERRANEAN DIET

The Mediterranean Diet is a dietary approach based on the traditional foods consumed by the people who inhabit the Mediterranean region. This diet has been studied and proven to have numerous health benefits, including reductions in risk for heart disease, stroke, cancer, and Alzheimer's disease, as well as improved longevity. It has also been shown to reduce the risk of obesity, diabetes, and metabolic syndrome. Additionally, there are benefits to mental health, including improved mood and cognitive function. The Mediterranean Diet is a well-balanced eating plan that focuses on fresh fruits and vegetables, whole grains, healthy fats, and lean proteins.

1. Reduced Risk of Heart Disease: Numerous studies have found that the Mediterranean Diet can reduce the risk of heart disease. This is due to the high intake of monounsaturated fats, such as olive oil, which are beneficial for heart health. The diet is also rich in omega-3 fatty acids, which have been shown to reduce the risk of heart disease. Additionally, the diet includes whole grains which are high in fiber, which helps to reduce cholesterol levels.

2. Reduced Risk of Stroke: The Mediterranean Diet is associated with a reduced risk of stroke due to its high intake of omega-3 fatty acids and monounsaturated fats. Additionally, the diet includes a variety of fruits and vegetables, which are high in antioxidants and can help to reduce inflammation and oxidative stress.

3. Reduced Risk of Cancer: Studies have found that the Mediterranean Diet can reduce the risk of certain types of cancer, such as colorectal, breast, and prostate cancer.

This is due to the high intake of fruits and vegetables, which are rich in antioxidants and can help to fight cancer-causing free radicals. Additionally, the diet includes healthy fats, such as olive oil, which can reduce inflammation and oxidative stress.

4. Reduced Risk of Alzheimer's Disease: Studies have found that the Mediterranean Diet can reduce the risk of Alzheimer's disease. This is due to the high intake of healthy fats, such as monounsaturated fats and omega-3 fatty acids. Additionally, the diet includes a variety of fruits and vegetables, which are high in antioxidants and can help to fight oxidative stress, which is a major risk factor for Alzheimer's.

5. Improved Longevity: Studies have found that the Mediterranean Diet can improve longevity by reducing the risk of numerous chronic diseases. This is due to the high intake of fruits and vegetables, which are rich in antioxidants and can help to fight free radicals.

Additionally, the diet includes healthy fats, such as olive oil, which can reduce inflammation and oxidative stress.

6. Reduced Risk of Obesity: The Mediterranean Diet is associated with a reduced risk of obesity due to its high intake of monounsaturated fats, fiber, and proteins. Additionally, the diet includes a variety of fresh fruits and vegetables, which are low in calories and can help to reduce calorie intake.

7. Reduced Risk of Diabetes: The Mediterranean Diet is associated with a reduced risk of diabetes due to its high intake of fiber, proteins, and healthy fats. Additionally, the diet includes a variety of fresh fruits and vegetables, which are low in calories and can help to reduce calorie intake.

8. Reduced Risk of Metabolic Syndrome: The Mediterranean Diet is associated with a reduced risk of metabolic syndrome due to its high intake of monounsaturated fats, fiber, and proteins.

Additionally, the diet includes a variety of fresh fruits and vegetables, which are low in calories and can help to reduce calorie intake.

9. Improved Mood: Studies have found that the Mediterranean Diet can improve mood due to its high intake of omega-3 fatty acids, which can help to reduce anxiety and depression. Additionally, the diet includes a variety of fresh fruits and vegetables, which are rich in antioxidants and can help to fight free radicals, which can contribute to mood disorders.

10. Improved Cognitive Function: The Mediterranean Diet is associated with improved cognitive function due to its high intake of omega-3 fatty acids and monounsaturated fats. Additionally, the diet includes a variety of fresh fruits and vegetables, which are rich in antioxidants and can help to fight free radicals, which can contribute to cognitive decline.

FOOD GROUPS OF THE MEDITERRANEAN DIET

The Mediterranean Diet is an eating pattern that is closely related with the traditional dietary patterns of the Mediterranean Sea's surrounding countries. It emphasizes the consumption of whole grains, fruits and vegetables, legumes, nuts and seeds, olive oil, and fish, while limiting the intake of red meat, dairy products, and processed foods. The Mediterranean Diet also encourages the consumption of herbs and spices, which are rich in antioxidants and other beneficial nutrients. This diet has been associated with numerous health benefits, including a reduced risk of obesity, heart disease, diabetes, and certain types of cancer.

The Mediterranean Diet is based on four main food groups:

1. Fruits and Vegetables: Fruits and vegetables are the foundation of the Mediterranean Diet.

They are low in calories and high in vitamins, minerals, fiber, and antioxidants. Aim to include at least 5 servings of fruits and vegetables in your daily diet.

2. Whole Grains: Whole grains provide essential vitamins, minerals, fiber, and other beneficial compounds. Choose whole grains such as oats, quinoa, brown rice, barley, and whole wheat bread and pasta.

3. Legumes, Nuts, and Seeds: Legumes, nuts, and seeds are excellent sources of protein, fiber, and healthy fats. Choose unsalted nuts and seeds, and legumes such as beans, lentils, and chickpeas.

4. Fish and Seafood: Fish and seafood are great sources of lean protein, omega-3 fatty acids, and other beneficial nutrients. Aim to include at least two servings of fish and seafood in your weekly diet.

GETTING STARTED ON A MEDITERRANEAN DIET

The Mediterranean Diet, or Med Diet, is a lifestyle that focuses on eating a variety of plant-based foods, such as vegetables, fruits, grains, and legumes, as well as healthy fats, lean proteins, and fish. This diet is often touted as a way to improve overall health and reduce the risk of chronic diseases, such as heart disease and diabetes. But many people don't know where to start when it comes to implementing a Med Diet. Here are some tips to get you started:

1. Eat plenty of fresh produce: Eating fresh fruits and veggies is the cornerstone of the Med Diet. Try to get at least five servings of fruits and vegetables each day. Choose a variety of colors, such as dark leafy greens, bright red tomatoes, and purple eggplants.

2. Include healthy fats: Healthy fats, such as olive oil, nuts, and seeds, are an important part of the Med Diet.

Use olive oil when cooking and eating salads, and try to include nuts or seeds in your meals.

3. Include lean proteins: Lean proteins, such as fish, poultry, and legumes, are an important part of the Med Diet. Aim for two to three servings of lean proteins each day.

4. Consider seafood: Seafood, such as salmon, mackerel, and sardines, are a part of the Med Diet. Aim for two to four servings of seafood each week.

5. Limit processed foods: Processed foods, such as refined grains, added sugars, and trans fats, should be limited as much as possible. Choose whole grains, such as quinoa or brown rice, when possible.

6. Enjoy meals with friends and family: Eating with others is an important part of the Med Diet. Share meals with friends and family, and take the time to enjoy your food.

7. Stay active: Physical activity is an important part of the Med Diet. Aim for at least 30 minutes of physical activity each day.

The Med Diet is a great way to eat for overall health and wellness. By following these tips, you'll be well on your way to a healthier lifestyle.

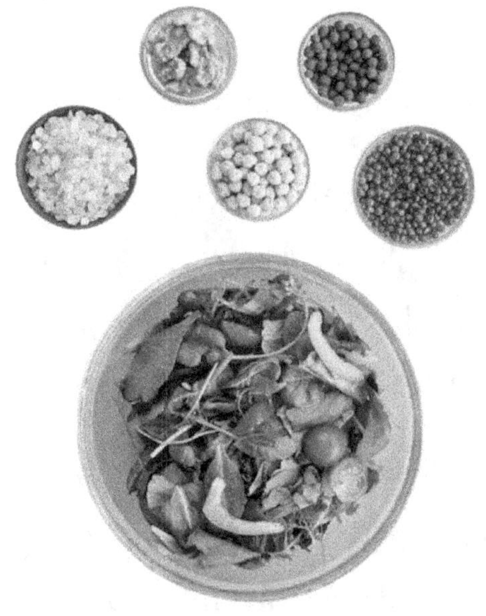

CHAPTER TWO

MEDITERRANEAN DIET BREAKFAST RECIPES

1. Mediterranean Granola Parfait

INGREDIENTS:

-1/4 cup rolled oats

-1/4 cup sliced almonds

-1/4 cup sunflower seeds

-1/4 cup pepitas

-2 tablespoons olive oil

-2 tablespoons honey

-1/4 teaspoon ground cinnamon

-1/4 cup Greek yogurt

-1/4 cup blueberries

-1/4 cup raspberries

-1/4 cup blackberries

INSTRUCTIONS:

1. Preheat oven to 350°F.

2. In a bowl, mix together the oats, almonds, sunflower seeds, and pepitas.

3. Drizzle with olive oil and honey, then sprinkle with cinnamon.

4. Spread the mixture out on a lined baking sheet.

5. Bake for 15 minutes, stirring halfway through.

6. Allow to cool before transferring to a bowl.

7. In a jar or glass, layer the yogurt, granola mixture, blueberries, raspberries, and blackberries.

8. Enjoy!

2. Mediterranean Egg Muffins

INGREDIENTS:

-2 tablespoons olive oil

-1/2 cup diced red bell pepper

-1/2 cup diced yellow onion

-1/2 cup diced spinach

-1/2 cup diced cherry tomatoes

-2 cloves garlic, minced

-1/2 teaspoon dried oregano

-1/2 teaspoon dried thyme

-1/4 teaspoon salt

-1/4 teaspoon freshly ground black pepper

-8 eggs

INSTRUCTIONS:

1. Preheat oven to 375°F.

2. Grease a 12-cup muffin tin with olive oil.

3. Heat the olive oil in a skillet over medium heat.

4. Add the bell pepper, onion, spinach, tomatoes, garlic, oregano, thyme, salt, and pepper.

5. Cook, stirring occasionally, until the vegetables are softened, about 5 minutes.

6. Divide the vegetable mixture among the muffin cups.

7. Crack an egg into each cup.

8. Bake for 20 minutes, or until the eggs are set.

9. Allow to cool before serving. Enjoy!

3. Greek Omelette

INGREDIENTS:

-2 tablespoons olive oil

-1/2 cup diced red onion

-1/2 cup diced red bell pepper

-1/2 cup diced zucchini

-1/2 cup crumbled feta cheese

-4 eggs

-Salt and freshly ground black pepper, to taste

INSTRUCTIONS:

1. Heat the olive oil in a skillet over medium heat.

2. Add the onion, bell pepper, and zucchini.

3. Cook, stirring occasionally, until the vegetables are softened, about 5 minutes.

4. In a bowl, whisk together the eggs, salt, and pepper.

5. Pour the egg mixture into the skillet.

6. Sprinkle the feta cheese over the top.

7. Cook until the eggs are set, about 5 minutes.

8. Flip the omelette and cook for an additional 3 minutes.

9. Slice and serve. Enjoy!

4. Mediterranean Toast

INGREDIENTS:

-2 slices whole wheat bread

-2 tablespoons olive oil

-2 tablespoons finely chopped fresh oregano

-2 tablespoons finely chopped fresh basil

-2 tablespoons finely chopped fresh parsley

-1/4 teaspoon salt

-1/4 teaspoon freshly ground black pepper

INSTRUCTIONS:

1. Preheat the oven to 350°F.

2. Place the bread slices on a baking sheet.

3. Drizzle with olive oil and sprinkle with oregano, basil, parsley, salt, and pepper.

4. Bake for 10 minutes, or until the bread is crispy.

5. Slice and serve. Enjoy!

5. Savory Greek Yogurt Bowl

INGREDIENTS:

-1 cup plain Greek yogurt

-2 tablespoons olive oil

-1/4 cup diced red onion

-1/4 cup diced cucumber

-1/4 cup diced tomato

-2 tablespoons chopped olives

-2 tablespoons crumbled feta cheese

-1 tablespoon freshly squeezed lemon juice

-Salt and freshly ground black pepper, to taste

INSTRUCTIONS:

1. In a bowl, mix together the yogurt, olive oil, red onion, cucumber, tomato, olives, feta, lemon juice, salt, and pepper.

2. Divide the mixture among two bowls.

3. Enjoy!

6. Mediterranean Quinoa Bowl

INGREDIENTS:

-1/2 cup uncooked quinoa

-1/2 cup diced tomatoes

-1/2 cup diced red onion

-1/2 cup diced zucchini

-1/2 cup diced yellow squash

-1/4 cup crumbled feta cheese

-2 tablespoons chopped olives

-2 tablespoons olive oil

-Salt and freshly ground black pepper, to taste

INSTRUCTIONS:

1. Cook the quinoa according to package instructions.

2. In a bowl, mix together the quinoa, tomatoes, onion, zucchini, squash, feta, olives, olive oil, salt, and pepper.

3. Divide the mixture among two bowls.

4. Enjoy!

7. Mediterranean Frittata

INGREDIENTS:

-2 tablespoons olive oil

-1/2 cup diced red onion

-1/2 cup diced red bell pepper

-1/2 cup diced zucchini

-1/2 cup diced yellow squash

-1/2 cup crumbled feta cheese

-4 eggs

-Salt and freshly ground black pepper, to taste

INSTRUCTIONS:

1. Preheat oven to 375°F.

2. Heat the olive oil in a skillet over medium heat.

3. Add the onion, bell pepper, zucchini, and squash.

4. Cook, stirring occasionally, until the vegetables are softened, about 5 minutes.

5. In a bowl, whisk together the eggs, salt, and pepper.

6. Pour the egg mixture into the skillet.

7. Sprinkle the feta cheese over the top.

8. Transfer the skillet to the oven and bake for 15 minutes, or until the eggs are set.

9. Slice and serve. Enjoy!

8. Mediterranean Toast with Avocado

INGREDIENTS:

-2 slices whole wheat bread

-1/2 avocado, mashed

-2 tablespoons olive oil

-2 tablespoons chopped fresh parsley

-1/4 teaspoon salt

-1/4 teaspoon freshly ground black pepper

INSTRUCTIONS:

1. Preheat the oven to 350°F.

2. Place the bread slices on a baking sheet.

3. Spread the mashed avocado on the bread slices.

4. Drizzle with olive oil and sprinkle with parsley, salt, and pepper.

5. Bake for 10 minutes, or until the bread is crispy.

6. Slice and serve. Enjoy!

9. Mediterranean Oatmeal Bowl

Ingredients:

-1/2 cup rolled oats

-2 tablespoons olive oil

-1/4 cup diced tomatoes

-1/4 cup diced red onion

-1/4 cup diced cucumber

-1/4 cup crumbled feta cheese

-2 tablespoons chopped olives

-1 tablespoon freshly squeezed lemon juice

-Salt and freshly ground black pepper, to taste

Instructions:

1. Cook the oatmeal according to package instructions.

2. In a bowl, mix together the oatmeal, olive oil, tomatoes, onion, cucumber, feta, olives, lemon juice, salt, and pepper.

3. Divide the mixture among two bowls.

4. Enjoy!

10. Mediterranean Breakfast Bowl

INGREDIENTS:

-1/2 cup uncooked quinoa

-2 tablespoons olive oil

-1/4 cup diced red bell pepper

-1/4 cup diced yellow onion

-1/4 cup diced zucchini

-1/4 cup diced cherry tomatoes

-2 tablespoons chopped olives

-2 tablespoons crumbled feta cheese

-1 tablespoon freshly squeezed lemon juice

-Salt and freshly ground black pepper, to taste

INSTRUCTIONS:

1. Cook the quinoa according to package instructions.

2. Heat the olive oil in a skillet over medium heat.

3. Add the bell pepper, onion, zucchini, and tomatoes.

4. Cook, stirring occasionally, until the vegetables are softened, about 5 minutes.

5. In a bowl, mix together the quinoa, vegetables, olives, feta, lemon juice, salt, and pepper.

6. Divide the mixture among two bowls.

7. Enjoy!

11. Mediterranean Egg Bake

INGREDIENTS:

-2 tablespoons olive oil

-1/2 cup diced red onion

-1/2 cup diced red bell pepper

-1/2 cup diced zucchini

-1/2 cup diced yellow squash

-1/2 cup crumbled feta cheese

-4 eggs

-Salt and freshly ground black pepper, to taste

INSTRUCTIONS:

1. Preheat oven to 375°F.

2. Heat the olive oil in a skillet over medium heat.

3. Add the onion, bell pepper, zucchini, and squash.

4. Cook, stirring occasionally, until the vegetables are softened, about 5 minutes.

5. Transfer the vegetables to an oven-safe baking dish.

6. In a bowl, whisk together the eggs, salt, and pepper.

7. Pour the egg mixture over the vegetables.

8. Sprinkle the feta cheese over the top.

9. Bake for 20 minutes, or until the eggs are set.

10. Slice and serve. Enjoy!

12. Mediterranean Omelette Wraps

INGREDIENTS:

-2 tablespoons olive oil

-1/2 cup diced red onion

-1/2 cup diced red bell pepper

-1/2 cup diced zucchini

-1/2 cup crumbled feta cheese

-4 eggs

-4 large lettuce leaves

-Salt and freshly ground black pepper, to taste

INSTRUCTIONS:

1. Heat the olive oil in a skillet over medium heat.

2. Add the onion, bell pepper, and zucchini.

3. Cook, stirring occasionally, until the vegetables are softened, about 5 minutes.

4. In a bowl, whisk together the eggs, salt, and pepper.

5. Pour the egg mixture into the skillet.

6. Sprinkle the feta cheese over the top.

7. Cook until the eggs are set, about 5 minutes.

8. Flip the omelette and cook for an additional 3 minutes.

9. Place the omelette on the lettuce leaves and wrap.

10. Slice and serve. Enjoy!

13. Mediterranean Yogurt Parfait

INGREDIENTS:

-1/2 cup plain Greek yogurt

-1/4 cup diced cucumber

-1/4 cup diced tomatoes

-2 tablespoons chopped olives

-2 tablespoons crumbled feta cheese

-1 tablespoon freshly squeezed lemon juice

-Salt and freshly ground black pepper, to taste

INSTRUCTIONS:

1. In a jar or glass, layer the yogurt, cucumber, tomatoes, olives, feta, and lemon juice.

2. Sprinkle with salt and pepper.

3. Enjoy!

14. Mediterranean Yogurt Bowl with Fruits

INGREDIENTS:

-1 cup plain Greek yogurt

-2 tablespoons olive oil

-1/4 cup diced red onion

-1/4 cup diced cucumber

-1/4 cup diced tomato

-2 tablespoons chopped olives

-2 tablespoons crumbled feta cheese

-1/4 cup diced pineapple

-1/4 cup diced mango

-1/4 cup diced strawberries

-1 tablespoon freshly squeezed lemon juice

-Salt and freshly ground black pepper, to taste

INSTRUCTIONS:

1. In a bowl, mix together the yogurt, olive oil, red onion, cucumber, tomato, olives, feta, pineapple, mango, strawberries, lemon juice, salt, and pepper.

2. Divide the mixture among two bowls.

3. Enjoy!

15. Mediterranean Smoothie Bowl

INGREDIENTS:

-1/2 cup plain Greek yogurt

-1/2 cup milk

-1/2 cup diced pineapple

-1/2 cup diced mango

-1/4 cup diced cucumber

-1/4 cup diced tomatoes

-2 tablespoons chopped olives

-2 tablespoons crumbled feta cheese

-1 tablespoon freshly squeezed lemon juice

-Salt and freshly ground black pepper, to taste

INSTRUCTIONS:

1. In a blender, combine the yogurt, milk, pineapple, mango, cucumber, tomatoes, olives, feta, lemon juice, salt, and pepper.

2. Blend until smooth.

3. Divide the mixture among two bowls.

4. Enjoy!

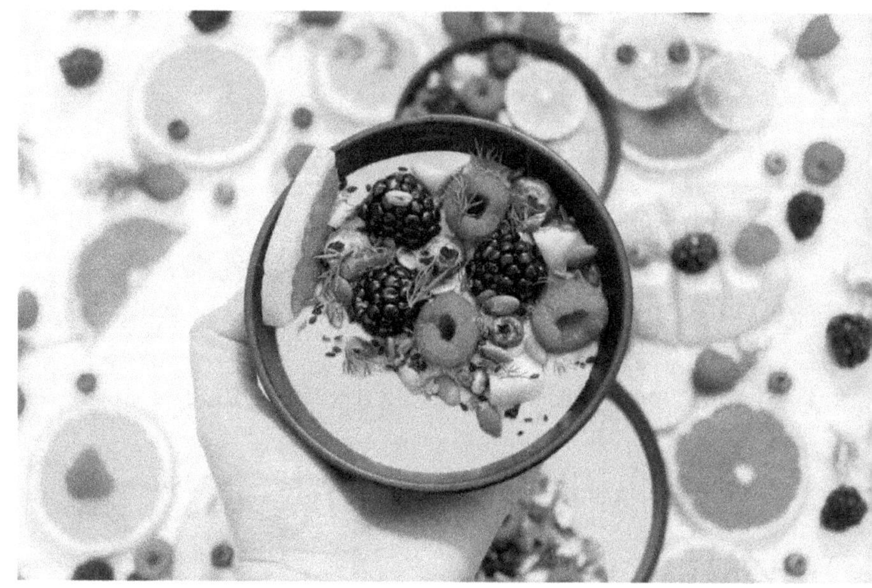

CHAPTER THREE

MEDITERRANEAN GRAIN, PASTA AND RICE RECIPES

1. Bulgur Wheat Salad with Chickpeas and Feta

INGREDIENTS:

- 2 cups bulgur wheat

- 1 can chickpeas, drained and rinsed

- 2 cups cherry tomatoes, quartered

- 1/2 cup diced red onion

- 1/2 cup crumbled feta cheese

- 2 tablespoons freshly chopped mint

- 2 tablespoons freshly chopped parsley

- 2 tablespoons freshly squeezed lemon juice

- 2 tablespoons olive oil

- Salt and pepper, to taste

INSTRUCTIONS:

1. Bring 2 cups of water to a boil in a medium pot.

2. Add the bulgur wheat and reduce heat to low. Simmer for 10 minutes, or until the bulgur is cooked through.

3. Drain any excess water, if needed, and transfer the bulgur to a large bowl.

4. Add the chickpeas, tomatoes, red onion, feta cheese, mint, and parsley to the bowl and stir to combine.

5. In a small bowl, whisk together the lemon juice, olive oil, salt, and pepper.

6. Pour the dressing over the salad and mix to combine.

7. Serve immediately or chill in the refrigerator for up to 2 days.

2. Mediterranean Farro Bowl

INGREDIENTS:

- 1 cup farro

- 1 bell pepper, chopped

- 1/2 cup black olives, pitted

- 1/2 cup feta cheese, crumbled

- 1/2 cup sun-dried tomatoes, chopped

- 2 tablespoons freshly chopped basil

- 2 tablespoons freshly chopped oregano

- 2 tablespoons olive oil

- 2 tablespoons freshly squeezed lemon juice

- Salt and pepper, to taste

INSTRUCTIONS:

1. Bring 2 cups of water to a boil in a medium pot.

2. Add the farro and reduce heat to low. Simmer for 10 minutes, or until the farro is cooked through.

3. Drain any excess water, if needed, and transfer the farro to a large bowl.

4. Add the bell pepper, olives, feta cheese, sun-dried tomatoes, basil, and oregano to the bowl and stir to combine.

5. In a small bowl, whisk together the olive oil, lemon juice, salt, and pepper.

6. Pour the dressing over the farro bowl and mix to combine.

7. Serve immediately or chill in the refrigerator for up to 2 days.

3. Mediterranean Rice Pilaf

INGREDIENTS:

- 2 cups long-grain white rice

- 1/2 cup diced red onion

- 1/2 cup diced bell pepper

- 1/2 cup sliced black olives

- 1/2 cup feta cheese, crumbled

- 2 tablespoons freshly chopped parsley

- 2 tablespoons freshly chopped oregano

- 2 tablespoons olive oil

- 2 tablespoons freshly squeezed lemon juice

- Salt and pepper, to taste

INSTRUCTIONS:

1. Bring 2 cups of water to a boil in a medium pot.

2. Add the rice and reduce heat to low. Simmer for 10 minutes, or until the rice is cooked through.

3. Drain any excess water, if needed, and transfer the rice to a large bowl.

4. Add the red onion, bell pepper, olives, feta cheese, parsley, and oregano to the bowl and stir to combine.

5. In a small bowl, whisk together the olive oil, lemon juice, salt, and pepper.

6. Pour the dressing over the rice pilaf and mix to combine.

7. Serve immediately or chill in the refrigerator for up to 2 days.

4. Mediterranean Quinoa Bowl

INGREDIENTS:

- 2 cups quinoa

- 1 can chickpeas, drained and rinsed

- 1/2 cup diced red onion

- 1/2 cup diced cucumber

- 1/2 cup crumbled feta cheese

- 2 tablespoons freshly chopped parsley

- 2 tablespoons freshly chopped mint

- 2 tablespoons olive oil

- 2 tablespoons freshly squeezed lemon juice

- Salt and pepper, to taste

INSTRUCTIONS:

1. Bring 2 cups of water to a boil in a medium pot.

2. Add the quinoa and reduce heat to low. Simmer for 10 minutes, or until the quinoa is cooked through.

3. Drain any excess water, if needed, and transfer the quinoa to a large bowl.

4. Add the chickpeas, red onion, cucumber, feta cheese, parsley, and mint to the bowl and stir to combine.

5. In a small bowl, whisk together the olive oil, lemon juice, salt, and pepper.

6. Pour the dressing over the quinoa bowl and mix to combine.

7. Serve immediately or chill in the refrigerator for up to 2 days.

5. Mediterranean Barley Salad

INGREDIENTS:

- 2 cups pearl barley

- 1 can chickpeas, drained and rinsed

- 1 cup cherry tomatoes, quartered

- 1/2 cup diced red onion

- 1/2 cup crumbled feta cheese

- 2 tablespoons freshly chopped parsley

- 2 tablespoons freshly chopped mint

- 2 tablespoons olive oil

- 2 tablespoons freshly squeezed lemon juice

- Salt and pepper, to taste

INSTRUCTIONS:

1. Bring 2 cups of water to a boil in a medium pot.

2. Add the barley and reduce heat to low. Simmer for 10 minutes, or until the barley is cooked through.

3. Drain any excess water, if needed, and transfer the barley to a large bowl.

4. Add the chickpeas, tomatoes, red onion, feta cheese, parsley, and mint to the bowl and stir to combine.

5. In a small bowl, whisk together the olive oil, lemon juice, salt, and pepper.

6. Pour the dressing over the barley salad and mix to combine.

7. Serve immediately or chill in the refrigerator for up to 2 days.

6. Mediterranean Orzo Salad

INGREDIENTS:

- 2 cups orzo

- 1 can chickpeas, drained and rinsed

- 1 cup cherry tomatoes, quartered

- 1/2 cup diced red onion

- 1/2 cup crumbled feta cheese

- 2 tablespoons freshly chopped parsley

- 2 tablespoons freshly chopped mint

- 2 tablespoons olive oil

- 2 tablespoons freshly squeezed lemon juice

- Salt and pepper, to taste

INSTRUCTIONS:

1. Bring 2 cups of water to a boil in a medium pot.

2. Add the orzo and reduce heat to low. Simmer for 10 minutes, or until the orzo is cooked through.

3. Drain any excess water, if needed, and transfer the orzo to a large bowl.

4. Add the chickpeas, tomatoes, red onion, feta cheese, parsley, and mint to the bowl and stir to combine.

5. In a small bowl, whisk together the olive oil, lemon juice, salt, and pepper.

6. Pour the dressing over the orzo salad and mix to combine.

7. Serve immediately or chill in the refrigerator for up to 2 days.

7. Mediterranean Couscous Salad

INGREDIENTS:

- 2 cups couscous

- 1 can chickpeas, drained and rinsed

- 1 cup cherry tomatoes, quartered

- 1/2 cup diced red onion

- 1/2 cup crumbled feta cheese

- 2 tablespoons freshly chopped parsley

- 2 tablespoons freshly chopped mint

- 2 tablespoons olive oil

- 2 tablespoons freshly squeezed lemon juice

- Salt and pepper, to taste

INSTRUCTIONS:

1. Bring 2 cups of water to a boil in a medium pot.

2. Add the couscous and reduce heat to low. Simmer for 10 minutes, or until the couscous is cooked through.

3. Drain any excess water, if needed, and transfer the couscous to a large bowl.

4. Add the chickpeas, tomatoes, red onion, feta cheese, parsley, and mint to the bowl and stir to combine.

5. In a small bowl, whisk together the olive oil, lemon juice, salt, and pepper.

6. Pour the dressing over the couscous salad and mix to combine.

7. Serve immediately or chill in the refrigerator for up to 2 days.

8. Mediterranean Freekeh Salad

INGREDIENTS:

- 2 cups freekeh

- 1 can chickpeas, drained and rinsed

- 1 cup cherry tomatoes, quartered

- 1/2 cup diced red onion

- 1/2 cup crumbled feta cheese

- 2 tablespoons freshly chopped parsley

- 2 tablespoons freshly chopped mint

- 2 tablespoons olive oil

- 2 tablespoons freshly squeezed lemon juice

- Salt and pepper, to taste

INSTRUCTIONS:

1. Bring 2 cups of water to a boil in a medium pot.

2. Add the freekeh and reduce heat to low. Simmer for 10 minutes, or until the freekeh is cooked through.

3. Drain any excess water, if needed, and transfer the freekeh to a large bowl.

4. Add the chickpeas, tomatoes, red onion, feta cheese, parsley, and mint to the bowl and stir to combine.

5. In a small bowl, whisk together the olive oil, lemon juice, salt, and pepper.

6. Pour the dressing over the freekeh salad and mix to combine.

7. Serve immediately or chill in the refrigerator for up to 2 days.

9. Mediterranean Bulgur Pilaf

INGREDIENTS:

- 2 cups bulgur wheat

- 1 can chickpeas, drained and rinsed

- 1/2 cup diced red onion

- 1/2 cup diced bell pepper

- 1/2 cup crumbled feta cheese

- 2 tablespoons freshly chopped parsley

- 2 tablespoons freshly chopped mint

- 2 tablespoons olive oil

- 2 tablespoons freshly squeezed lemon juice

- Salt and pepper, to taste

INSTRUCTIONS:

1. Bring 2 cups of water to a boil in a medium pot.

2. Add the bulgur wheat and reduce heat to low. Simmer for 10 minutes, or until the bulgur is cooked through.

3. Drain any excess water, if needed, and transfer the bulgur to a large bowl.

4. Add the chickpeas, red onion, bell pepper, feta cheese, parsley, and mint to the bowl and stir to combine.

5. In a small bowl, whisk together the olive oil, lemon juice, salt, and pepper.

6. Pour the dressing over the bulgur pilaf and mix to combine.

7. Serve immediately or chill in the refrigerator for up to 2 days.

10. Mediterranean Lentil Salad

INGREDIENTS:

- 2 cups lentils

- 1 can chickpeas, drained and rinsed

- 1 cup cherry tomatoes, quartered

- 1/2 cup diced red onion

- 1/2 cup crumbled feta cheese

- 2 tablespoons freshly chopped parsley

- 2 tablespoons freshly chopped mint

- 2 tablespoons olive oil

- 2 tablespoons freshly squeezed lemon juice

- Salt and pepper, to taste

INSTRUCTIONS:

1. Bring 2 cups of water to a boil in a medium pot.

2. Add the lentils and reduce heat to low. Simmer for 10 minutes, or until the lentils are cooked through.

3. Drain any excess water, if needed, and transfer the lentils to a large bowl.

4. Add the chickpeas, tomatoes, red onion, feta cheese, parsley, and mint to the bowl and stir to combine.

5. In a small bowl, whisk together the olive oil, lemon juice, salt, and pepper.

6. Pour the dressing over the lentil salad and mix to combine.

7. Serve immediately or chill in the refrigerator for up to 2 days.

CHAPTER FOUR

MEDITERRANEAN VEGETABLE & BEAN RECIPES

1. Roasted Eggplant and Chickpea Salad

INGREDIENTS:

- 2 large eggplants, cubed

- 2 cups cooked chickpeas

- 2 cloves garlic, minced

- 2 tablespoons olive oil

- 1 teaspoon ground cumin

- Salt and pepper to taste

- 2 tablespoons freshly chopped parsley

- 2 tablespoons freshly chopped mint

- 1/4 cup crumbled feta cheese

INSTRUCTIONS:

- Preheat oven to 400°F.

- Place the cubed eggplant on a baking sheet and drizzle with 1 tablespoon of the olive oil.

- Sprinkle with a pinch of salt and pepper, then roast for 20 minutes.

- In a large bowl, mix together the cooked chickpeas, garlic, cumin, remaining tablespoon of olive oil, salt and pepper.

- Add the roasted eggplant to the bowl and mix until combined.

- Garnish with parsley, mint, and feta cheese.

- Serve warm or chilled.

2. Mediterranean White Bean Soup

INGREDIENTS:

- 2 tablespoons olive oil

- 1 onion, diced

- 2 cloves garlic, minced

- 2 carrots, diced

- 2 celery stalks, diced

- 2 teaspoons dried oregano

- 2 teaspoons dried thyme

- 6 cups vegetable broth

- 2 cans (15 ounces each) white beans, drained and rinsed

- 1/4 cup freshly chopped parsley

- Salt and pepper to taste

INSTRUCTIONS:

- Heat the olive oil in a large pot over medium heat.

- Add the onion, garlic, carrots, and celery and cook until softened, about 5 minutes.

- Add the oregano and thyme and cook for another minute.

- Add the vegetable broth and white beans and bring to a boil.

- Reduce the heat and simmer for 15 minutes.

- Stir in the parsley and season with salt and pepper to taste.

- Serve warm.

3. Mediterranean Roasted Vegetable and Bean Salad

INGREDIENTS:

- 2 large sweet potatoes, cubed

- 1 red bell pepper, chopped

- 1 yellow bell pepper, chopped

- 1 red onion, chopped

- 2 tablespoons olive oil

- 2 cloves garlic, minced

- 1 teaspoon dried oregano

- 1 teaspoon dried thyme

- 2 cans (15 ounces each) black beans, drained and rinsed

- 2 tablespoons freshly chopped parsley

- 2 tablespoons freshly chopped basil

- 2 tablespoons freshly chopped mint

- 1/4 cup crumbled feta cheese

- Salt and pepper to taste

INSTRUCTIONS:

- Preheat oven to 400°F.

- Place the cubed sweet potatoes, bell peppers, and red onion on a baking sheet and drizzle with 1 tablespoon of the olive oil.

- Sprinkle with a pinch of salt and pepper, then roast for 20 minutes.

- In a large bowl, mix together the cooked black beans, garlic, oregano, thyme, remaining tablespoon of olive oil, salt and pepper.

- Add the roasted vegetables to the bowl and mix until combined.

- Garnish with parsley, basil, mint, and feta cheese.

- Serve warm or chilled.

4. Mediterranean Lentil Soup

INGREDIENTS:

- 2 tablespoons olive oil

- 1 onion, diced

- 2 cloves garlic, minced

- 2 carrots, diced

- 2 celery stalks, diced

- 1 teaspoon ground cumin

- 2 teaspoons dried oregano

- 1 teaspoon dried thyme

- 6 cups vegetable broth

- 1 cup dried lentils

- 2 cans (15 ounces each) diced tomatoes

- 2 tablespoons freshly chopped parsley

- Salt and pepper to taste

INSTRUCTIONS:

- Heat the olive oil in a large pot over medium heat.

- Add the onion, garlic, carrots, and celery and cook until softened, about 5 minutes.

- Add the cumin, oregano, and thyme and cook for another minute.

- Add the vegetable broth, lentils, and diced tomatoes and bring to a boil.

- Reduce the heat and simmer for 25 minutes.

- Stir in the parsley and season with salt and pepper to taste.

- Serve warm.

5. Mediterranean Baked Beans

INGREDIENTS:

- 2 tablespoons olive oil

- 1 onion, diced

- 2 cloves garlic, minced

- 2 cans (15 ounces each) white beans, drained and rinsed

- 1 cup vegetable broth

- 2 tablespoons tomato paste

- 1 teaspoon dried oregano

- 1 teaspoon dried thyme

- 2 tablespoons freshly chopped parsley

- 2 tablespoons freshly chopped basil

- 2 tablespoons freshly chopped mint

- Salt and pepper to taste

INSTRUCTIONS:

- Preheat oven to 350°F.

- Heat the olive oil in a large pot over medium heat.

- Add the onion and garlic and cook until softened, about 5 minutes.

- Add the white beans, vegetable broth, tomato paste, oregano, thyme, salt, and pepper and bring to a boil.

- Reduce the heat and simmer for 10 minutes.

- Transfer the bean mixture to a baking dish and sprinkle with the parsley, basil, and mint.

- Bake for 30 minutes.

- Serve warm.

6. Mediterranean Bean Burgers

INGREDIENTS:

- 2 cans (15 ounces each) black beans, drained and rinsed

- 1/2 cup cooked quinoa

- 1/2 cup rolled oats

- 1/4 cup crumbled feta cheese

- 2 tablespoons freshly chopped parsley

- 2 tablespoons freshly chopped basil

- 2 tablespoons freshly chopped mint

- 2 cloves garlic, minced

- 1 teaspoon ground cumin

- 1 teaspoon dried oregano

- 2 tablespoons olive oil

- Salt and pepper to taste

INSTRUCTIONS:

- In a large bowl, mash the beans using a fork or potato masher.

- Add the cooked quinoa, rolled oats, feta cheese, parsley, basil, mint, garlic, cumin, oregano, olive oil, salt, and pepper and mix until combined.

- Form the mixture into 4 patties.

- Heat a large skillet over medium heat and add the patties.

- Cook until golden brown and crispy, about 5 minutes per side.

- Serve with your favorite toppings.

7. Mediterranean Stuffed Peppers

INGREDIENTS:

- 4 large bell peppers, halved and seeded

- 2 tablespoons olive oil

- 1 onion, diced

- 2 cloves garlic, minced

- 1 teaspoon ground cumin

- 2 teaspoons dried oregano

- 2 cans (15 ounces each) white beans, drained and rinsed

- 1/2 cup cooked quinoa

- 1 cup tomato sauce

- 2 tablespoons freshly chopped parsley

- 2 tablespoons freshly chopped basil

- 2 tablespoons freshly chopped mint

- 1/4 cup crumbled feta cheese

- Salt and pepper to taste

INSTRUCTIONS:

- Preheat oven to 400°F.

- Place the bell pepper halves in a baking dish and drizzle with 1 tablespoon of the olive oil.

- Roast for 20 minutes.

- Heat the remaining tablespoon of olive oil in a large skillet over medium heat.

- Add the onion, garlic, cumin, and oregano and cook until softened, about 5 minutes.

- Add the white beans, cooked quinoa, tomato sauce, parsley, basil, mint, salt, and pepper and cook for another 5 minutes.

- Fill the roasted bell peppers with the bean mixture and top with feta cheese.

- Bake for 15 minutes.

- Serve warm.

8. Mediterranean Vegetable Stew

INGREDIENTS:

- 2 tablespoons olive oil

- 1 onion, diced

- 2 cloves garlic, minced

- 2 carrots, diced

- 2 celery stalks, diced

- 2 teaspoons dried oregano

- 2 teaspoons dried thyme

- 6 cups vegetable broth

- 1 zucchini, cubed

- 1 yellow squash, cubed

- 1 eggplant, cubed

- 2 cans (15 ounces each) white beans, drained and rinsed

- 2 tablespoons freshly chopped parsley

- Salt and pepper to taste

INSTRUCTIONS:

- Heat the olive oil in a large pot over medium heat.

- Add the onion, garlic, carrots, and celery and cook until softened, about 5 minutes.

- Add the oregano and thyme and cook for another minute.

- Add the vegetable broth, zucchini, yellow squash, eggplant, and white beans and bring to a boil.

- Reduce the heat and simmer for 20 minutes.

- Stir in the parsley and season with salt and pepper to taste.

- Serve warm.

9. Mediterranean Baked Beans with Spinach

INGREDIENTS:

- 2 tablespoons olive oil

- 1 onion, diced

- 2 cloves garlic, minced

- 2 cans (15 ounces each) white beans, drained and rinsed

- 1 cup vegetable broth

- 2 tablespoons tomato paste

- 1 teaspoon dried oregano

- 1 teaspoon dried thyme

- 2 cups fresh spinach

- 2 tablespoons freshly chopped parsley

- 2 tablespoons freshly chopped basil

- 2 tablespoons freshly chopped mint

- Salt and pepper to taste

INSTRUCTIONS:

- Preheat oven to 350°F.

- Heat the olive oil in a large pot over medium heat.

- Add the onion and garlic and cook until softened, about 5 minutes.

- Add the white beans, vegetable broth, tomato paste, oregano, thyme, salt, and pepper and bring to a boil.

- Reduce the heat and simmer for 10 minutes.

- Add the spinach and stir until wilted.

- Transfer the bean mixture to a baking dish and sprinkle with the parsley, basil, and mint.

- Bake for 30 minutes.

- Serve warm.

10. Mediterranean Chickpea Salad

INGREDIENTS:

- 2 cans (15 ounces each) chickpeas, drained and rinsed

- 2 cloves garlic, minced

- 2 tablespoons olive oil

- 1 teaspoon ground cumin

- 2 tablespoons freshly chopped parsley

- 2 tablespoons freshly chopped mint

- 1/4 cup crumbled feta cheese

- Salt and pepper to taste

INSTRUCTIONS:

- In a large bowl, mix together the chickpeas, garlic, olive oil, cumin, salt, and pepper.

- Add the parsley, mint, and feta cheese and mix until combined.

- Serve chilled or at room temperature.

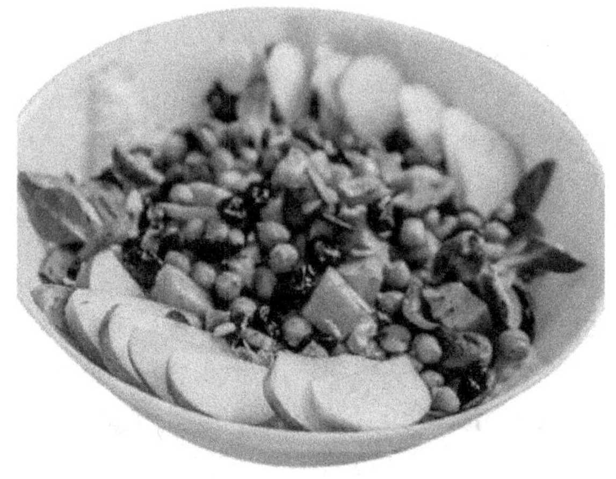

CHAPTER FIVE

MEDITERRANEAN SEAFOOD AND FISH

1. Mediterranean Baked Salmon

INGREDIENTS:

- 4 (4-6 ounce) salmon fillets

- 2 tablespoons olive oil

- 2 tablespoons freshly squeezed lemon juice

- 2 cloves garlic, minced

- 1 teaspoon dried oregano

- 1/2 teaspoon dried thyme

- Salt and freshly ground black pepper, to taste

INSTRUCTIONS:

1. Preheat oven to 400°F.

2. Place salmon fillets in a baking dish.

3. In a small bowl, whisk together olive oil, lemon juice, garlic, oregano, and thyme; season with salt and pepper, to taste.

4. Pour the olive oil mixture over the salmon fillets.

5. Bake in preheated oven until the fish is cooked through, about 15-20 minutes.

2. Grilled Mediterranean Sea Bass

INGREDIENTS:

- 4 (4-6 ounce) sea bass fillets

- 2 tablespoons olive oil

- 2 tablespoons freshly squeezed lemon juice

- 2 cloves garlic, minced

- 1 teaspoon dried oregano

- 1/2 teaspoon dried thyme

- Salt and freshly ground black pepper, to taste

INSTRUCTIONS:

1. Preheat a grill to medium-high heat.

2. Brush the sea bass fillets with olive oil, then season with lemon juice, garlic, oregano, thyme, salt, and pepper, to taste.

3. Place the fillets on the preheated grill, and cook until the fish is cooked through, about 3-4 minutes per side.

3. Mediterranean Shrimp Skewers

INGREDIENTS:

- 1 pound shrimp, peeled and deveined

- 2 tablespoons olive oil

- 2 cloves garlic, minced

- 2 tablespoons freshly squeezed lemon juice

- 1 teaspoon dried oregano

- 1/2 teaspoon dried thyme

- Salt and freshly ground black pepper, to taste

INSTRUCTIONS:

1. Preheat a grill or a grill pan to medium-high heat.

2. In a small bowl, whisk together olive oil, garlic, lemon juice, oregano, thyme, salt, and pepper; pour over shrimp and toss to coat.

3. Thread the shrimp onto skewers, about 4-5 per skewer.

4. Place the skewers onto the preheated grill and cook until the shrimp are opaque and cooked through, about 2-3 minutes per side.

4. Mediterranean Tuna Fettuccine

INGREDIENTS:

- 8 ounces fettuccine

- 2 tablespoons olive oil

- 1 (7-ounce) can tuna, drained

- 2 cloves garlic, minced

- 2 tablespoons capers

- 2 tablespoons freshly squeezed lemon juice

- 1 teaspoon dried oregano

- 1/2 teaspoon dried thyme

- Salt and freshly ground black pepper, to taste

INSTRUCTIONS:

1. Cook the fettuccine according to package instructions; drain well.

2. In a large skillet over medium heat, heat olive oil.

3. Add tuna, garlic, capers, lemon juice, oregano, thyme, salt, and pepper; cook, stirring occasionally, until heated through, about 3-4 minutes.

4. Add the cooked fettuccine and toss to combine; cook, stirring occasionally, for 2-3 minutes.

5. Mediterranean Mussels

INGREDIENTS:

- 2 pounds mussels

- 2 tablespoons olive oil

- 2 cloves garlic, minced

- 1/2 cup white wine

- 2 tablespoons freshly squeezed lemon juice

- 1 teaspoon dried oregano

- 1/2 teaspoon dried thyme

- Salt and freshly ground black pepper, to taste

INSTRUCTIONS:

1. In a large pot over medium heat, heat olive oil.

2. Add garlic, white wine, lemon juice, oregano, thyme, salt, and pepper; bring to a boil.

3. Add the mussels, cover, and cook for about 8-10 minutes, or until the mussels open. Discard any mussels that do not open.

4. Serve the mussels warm with the cooking liquid.

6. Mediterranean Grilled Octopus

INGREDIENTS:

- 2 pounds octopus, cleaned and cut into pieces

- 2 tablespoons olive oil

- 2 cloves garlic, minced

- 2 tablespoons freshly squeezed lemon juice

- 1 teaspoon dried oregano

- 1/2 teaspoon dried thyme

- Salt and freshly ground black pepper, to taste

INSTRUCTIONS:

1. Preheat a grill or a grill pan to medium-high heat.

2. Brush the octopus with olive oil, then season with garlic, lemon juice, oregano, thyme, salt, and pepper, to taste.

3. Place the octopus pieces on the preheated grill and cook until lightly charred and cooked through, about 3-4 minutes per side.

7.   Mediterranean   Calamari Salad

INGREDIENTS:

- 1 pound calamari, cleaned and cut into rings

- 2 tablespoons olive oil

- 2 cloves garlic, minced

- 2 tablespoons freshly squeezed lemon juice

- 1 teaspoon dried oregano

- 1/2 teaspoon dried thyme

- Salt and freshly ground black pepper, to taste

- 1/2 cup chopped fresh parsley

- 2 tablespoons capers

- 1/4 cup diced red onion

INSTRUCTIONS:

1. In a large skillet over medium heat, heat olive oil.

2. Add garlic, lemon juice, oregano, thyme, salt, and pepper; cook, stirring occasionally, until fragrant, about 1-2 minutes.

3. Add the calamari rings and cook until lightly browned and cooked through, about 3-4 minutes.

4. Remove from heat and let cool slightly.

5. In a large bowl, combine the cooked calamari, parsley, capers, and red onion.

6. Serve the salad warm or at room temperature.

8. Mediterranean Stuffed Clams

INGREDIENTS:

- 24 clams

- 2 tablespoons olive oil

- 2 cloves garlic, minced

- 2 tablespoons freshly squeezed lemon juice

- 1 teaspoon dried oregano

- 1/2 teaspoon dried thyme

- Salt and freshly ground black pepper, to taste

- 1/2 cup Italian-style breadcrumbs

- 1/4 cup grated Parmesan cheese

INSTRUCTIONS:

1. Preheat oven to 400°F.

2. In a large skillet over medium heat, heat olive oil.

3. Add garlic, lemon juice, oregano, thyme, salt, and pepper; cook, stirring occasionally, until fragrant, about 1-2 minutes.

4. Remove from heat and let cool slightly.

5. In a large bowl, combine the breadcrumbs, Parmesan cheese, and cooled garlic mixture.

6. Stuff the mixture into the clams, then place the clams onto a baking sheet.

7. Bake in preheated oven until the clams are cooked through, about 10-12 minutes.

9. Mediterranean Baked Cod

INGREDIENTS:

- 4 (4-6 ounce) cod fillets

- 2 tablespoons olive oil

- 2 tablespoons freshly squeezed lemon juice

- 2 cloves garlic, minced

- 1 teaspoon dried oregano

- 1/2 teaspoon dried thyme

- Salt and freshly ground black pepper, to taste

INSTRUCTIONS:

1. Preheat oven to 400°F.

2. Place cod fillets in a baking dish.

3. In a small bowl, whisk together olive oil, lemon juice, garlic, oregano, and thyme; season with salt and pepper, to taste.

4. Pour the olive oil mixture over the cod fillets.

5. Bake in preheated oven until the fish is cooked through, about 15-20 minutes.

10.   Mediterranean   Grilled Sardines

INGREDIENTS:

- 4 (4-6 ounce) sardines

- 2 tablespoons olive oil

- 2 tablespoons freshly squeezed lemon juice

- 2 cloves garlic, minced

- 1 teaspoon dried oregano

- 1/2 teaspoon dried thyme

- Salt and freshly ground black pepper, to taste

INSTRUCTIONS:

1. Preheat a grill or a grill pan to medium-high heat.

2. Brush the sardines with olive oil, then season with lemon juice, garlic, oregano, thyme, salt, and pepper, to taste.

3. Place the sardines onto the preheated grill and cook until lightly charred and cooked through, about 3-4 minutes per side.

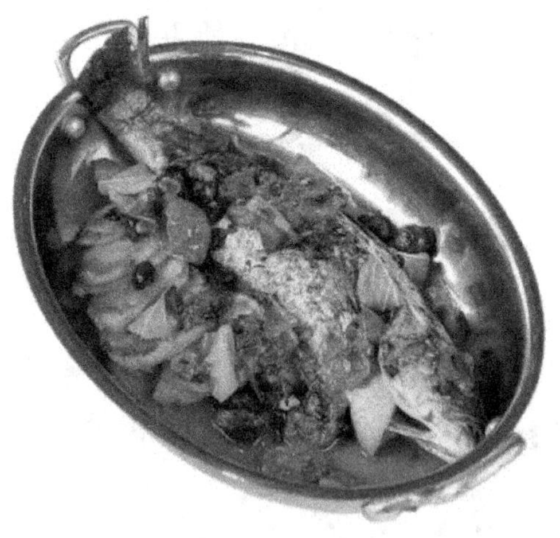

CHAPTER SIX

MEDITERRANEAN MEAT AND POULTRY RECIPES

1. Grilled Lamb Chops with Garlic and Oregano

INGREDIENTS:

- 8 lamb chops

- 4 cloves garlic, minced

- 2 tablespoons fresh oregano, chopped

- 2 tablespoons olive oil

- Salt and pepper, to taste

INSTRUCTIONS:

- Preheat the grill to medium-high heat.

- In a medium bowl, mix together garlic, oregano, olive oil, salt, and pepper.

- Rub the mixture over the lamb chops.

- Place the lamb chops on the grill and cook for about 5 minutes per side, or until cooked through.

- Serve with your favorite sides.

2. Greek Roasted Chicken

INGREDIENTS:

- 1 whole chicken, cut into 8 pieces

- 2 tablespoons olive oil

- 1 teaspoon garlic powder

- 1 teaspoon dried oregano

- 1 teaspoon dried thyme

- Salt and pepper, to taste

INSTRUCTIONS:

- Preheat the oven to 400°F.

- Place the chicken pieces in a large baking dish.

- Drizzle with olive oil and sprinkle with garlic powder, oregano, thyme, salt, and pepper.

- Bake for 40 minutes, or until the chicken is cooked through.

- Serve with your favorite sides.

3. Baked Falafel

INGREDIENTS:

- 2 cans chickpeas, drained and rinsed

- 1/2 onion, finely chopped

- 2 cloves garlic, minced

- 2 tablespoons fresh parsley, chopped

- 2 tablespoons fresh cilantro, chopped

- 2 tablespoons all-purpose flour

- 1 teaspoon ground cumin

- 1 teaspoon ground coriander

- 1/4 teaspoon baking soda

- Salt and pepper, to taste

INSTRUCTIONS:

- Preheat the oven to 350°F.

- In a food processor, combine the chickpeas, onion, garlic, parsley, cilantro, flour, cumin, coriander, baking soda, salt, and pepper. Pulse until everything is finely chopped and the mixture is combined.

- Form the mixture into small balls and place on a baking sheet.

- Bake for 20 minutes, or until the falafel are golden brown.

- Serve with hummus, tzatziki, or your favorite sauce.

4. Baked Stuffed Chicken Breasts

INGREDIENTS:

- 4 boneless, skinless chicken breasts

- 1 cup spinach leaves, chopped

- 1/2 cup feta cheese, crumbled

- 2 cloves garlic, minced

- 2 tablespoons olive oil

- Salt and pepper, to taste

INSTRUCTIONS:

- Preheat the oven to 350°F.

- Place the chicken breasts in a baking dish.

- In a medium bowl, mix together the spinach, feta, garlic, olive oil, salt, and pepper.

- Stuff the chicken breasts with the spinach mixture.

- Bake for 30 minutes, or until the chicken is cooked through.

- Serve with your favorite sides.

5. Grilled Turkey Kebabs

INGREDIENTS:

- 1 pound ground turkey

- 1/2 onion, diced

- 2 cloves garlic, minced

- 2 tablespoons fresh parsley, chopped

- 2 tablespoons olive oil

- 1 teaspoon ground cumin

- 1 teaspoon ground coriander

- Salt and pepper, to taste

INSTRUCTIONS:

- Preheat the grill to medium-high heat.

- In a medium bowl, mix together the ground turkey, onion, garlic, parsley, olive oil, cumin, coriander, salt, and pepper.

- Form the mixture into 8 kebab patties.

- Grill the kebabs for about 5 minutes per side, or until cooked through.

- Serve with your favorite sides.

6. Greek Baked Pork Chops

INGREDIENTS:

- 4 pork chops

- 2 tablespoons olive oil

- 2 cloves garlic, minced

- 2 tablespoons fresh oregano, chopped

- 2 tablespoons fresh thyme, chopped

- Salt and pepper, to taste

INSTRUCTIONS:

- Preheat the oven to 400°F.

- Place the pork chops in a baking dish.

- Drizzle with olive oil and sprinkle with garlic, oregano, thyme, salt, and pepper.

- Bake for 25 minutes, or until the pork is cooked through.

- Serve with your favorite sides.

7. Greek Chicken Souvlaki

INGREDIENTS:

- 1 pound boneless, skinless chicken breasts, cut into 1-inch cubes

- 2 tablespoons olive oil

- 2 cloves garlic, minced

- 2 tablespoons fresh oregano, chopped

- 2 tablespoons fresh thyme, chopped

- Salt and pepper, to taste

INSTRUCTIONS:

- Preheat the grill to medium-high heat.

- In a medium bowl, mix together the chicken, olive oil, garlic, oregano, thyme, salt, and pepper.

- Thread the chicken onto skewers and place on the grill.

- Grill for about 5 minutes per side, or until the chicken is cooked through.

- Serve with your favorite sides.

8. Mediterranean Turkey Burgers

INGREDIENTS:

- 1 pound ground turkey

- 1/2 onion, diced

- 2 cloves garlic, minced

- 2 tablespoons fresh parsley, chopped

- 2 tablespoons olive oil

- 1 teaspoon ground cumin

- 1 teaspoon ground coriander

- Salt and pepper, to taste

INSTRUCTIONS:

- Preheat the grill to medium-high heat.

- In a medium bowl, mix together the ground turkey, onion, garlic, parsley, olive oil, cumin, coriander, salt, and pepper.

- Form the mixture into 4 patties.

- Grill the burgers for about 5 minutes per side, or until cooked through.

- Serve on buns with your favorite toppings.

9. Grilled Spiced Chicken

INGREDIENTS:

- 4 boneless, skinless chicken breasts

- 1/4 cup olive oil

- 2 cloves garlic, minced

- 2 tablespoons fresh oregano, chopped

- 2 tablespoons fresh thyme, chopped

- 1 teaspoon ground cumin

- 1 teaspoon ground coriander

- Salt and pepper, to taste

INSTRUCTIONS:

- Preheat the grill to medium-high heat.

- In a medium bowl, mix together the olive oil, garlic, oregano, thyme, cumin, coriander, salt, and pepper.

- Rub the mixture over the chicken breasts.

- Place the chicken on the grill and cook for about 5 minutes per side, or until cooked through.

- Serve with your favorite sides.

10. Mediterranean Stuffed Peppers

INGREDIENTS:

- 4 bell peppers, halved and seeded

- 1/2 pound ground turkey

- 1/2 onion, diced

- 2 cloves garlic, minced

- 2 tablespoons fresh parsley, chopped

- 2 tablespoons olive oil

- 1 teaspoon ground cumin

- 1 teaspoon ground coriander

- Salt and pepper, to taste

INSTRUCTIONS:

- Preheat the oven to 350°F.

- In a medium bowl, mix together the ground turkey, onion, garlic, parsley, olive oil, cumin, coriander, salt, and pepper.

- Stuff the pepper halves with the turkey mixture.

- Place the peppers in a baking dish and bake for 30 minutes, or until the peppers are tender and the turkey is cooked through.

- Serve with your favorite sides.

9.   Mediterranean   Stuffed Peppers

INGREDIENTS:

- 4 bell peppers, halved and seeded

- 1/2 pound ground turkey

- 1/2 onion, diced

- 2 cloves garlic, minced

- 2 tablespoons fresh parsley, chopped

- 2 tablespoons olive oil

- 1 teaspoon ground cumin

- 1 teaspoon ground coriander

- Salt and pepper, to taste

INSTRUCTIONS:

- Preheat the oven to 350°F.

- In a medium bowl, mix together the ground turkey, onion, garlic, parsley, olive oil, cumin, coriander, salt, and pepper.

- Stuff the pepper halves with the turkey mixture.

- Place the peppers in a baking dish and bake for 30 minutes, or until the peppers are tender and the turkey is cooked through.

- Serve with your favorite sides.

10.   Mediterranean   Roasted Turkey Breast

INGREDIENTS:

- 1 turkey breast

- 2 tablespoons olive oil

- 2 cloves garlic, minced

- 2 tablespoons fresh oregano, chopped

- 2 tablespoons fresh thyme, chopped

- Salt and pepper, to taste

INSTRUCTIONS:

- Preheat the oven to 375°F.

- Place the turkey breast in a baking dish.

- Drizzle with olive oil and sprinkle with garlic, oregano, thyme, salt, and pepper.

- Bake for 1 hour, or until the turkey is cooked through.

- Serve with your favorite sides.

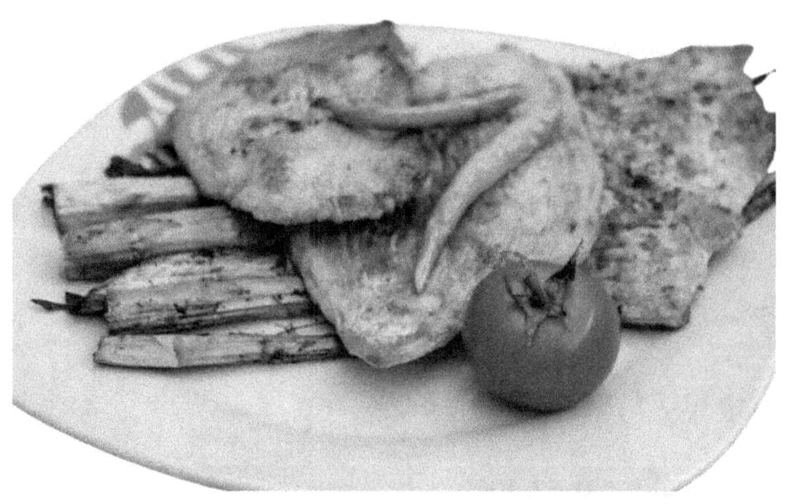

CHAPTER SEVEN

MEDITERRANEAN SALAD RECIPES

1. Mediterranean Grilled Chicken Salad

INGREDIENTS:

- 2 boneless skinless chicken breasts

- 2 tablespoons olive oil

- Salt and pepper to taste

- 2 cups baby spinach

- 2 cups arugula

- 1/2 cup cherry tomatoes, halved

- 1/2 cup cucumber, diced

- 1/2 cup kalamata olives, pitted and halved

- 1/4 cup feta cheese, crumbled

- 2 tablespoons fresh parsley, finely chopped

- 2 tablespoons red wine vinegar

- 2 tablespoons olive oil

INSTRUCTIONS:

1. Preheat a grill or grill pan to medium heat.

2. Rub the chicken breasts with 2 tablespoons of olive oil and season with salt and pepper to taste.

3. Place chicken on the grill and cook for 4-5 minutes per side, or until cooked through.

4. Remove chicken from the grill and let rest for 5 minutes before slicing into strips.

5. In a large bowl, combine the spinach, arugula, tomatoes, cucumber, olives, feta cheese, and parsley.

6. In a separate bowl, whisk together the red wine vinegar, olive oil, salt, and pepper.

7. Pour the dressing over the salad and toss to combine.

8. Top the salad with the grilled chicken strips.

9. Serve and enjoy!

2. Mediterranean Couscous Salad

INGREDIENTS:

- 2 cups couscous

- 2 cups vegetable broth

- 2 tablespoons olive oil

- 2 tablespoons lemon juice

- 1 teaspoon garlic powder

- 1/2 teaspoon oregano

- 1/4 teaspoon red pepper flakes

- 1/2 cup cherry tomatoes, halved

- 1/2 cup cucumber, diced

- 1/2 cup kalamata olives, pitted and halved

- 1/4 cup feta cheese, crumbled

- 2 tablespoons fresh parsley, finely chopped

INSTRUCTIONS:

1. Bring the vegetable broth to a boil in a medium saucepan.

2. Stir in the couscous and reduce heat to low.

3. Cover and cook for 8-10 minutes, or until the couscous is tender.

4. Remove from heat and fluff with a fork.

5. In a small bowl, whisk together the olive oil, lemon juice, garlic powder, oregano, and red pepper flakes.

6. In a large bowl, combine the cooked couscous, tomatoes, cucumber, olives, feta cheese, and parsley.

7. Pour the dressing over the salad and toss to combine.

8. Serve and enjoy!

3. Mediterranean Chopped Salad

INGREDIENTS:

- 2 cups chopped romaine lettuce

- 2 cups chopped spinach

- 1 cup diced red bell pepper

- 1 cup diced cucumber

- 1/2 cup diced red onion

- 1/2 cup diced kalamata olives

- 1/4 cup feta cheese, crumbled

- 2 tablespoons fresh parsley, finely chopped

- 2 tablespoons olive oil

- 2 tablespoons red wine vinegar

- 2 teaspoons honey

- 1/2 teaspoon garlic powder

- 1/4 teaspoon oregano

- 1/4 teaspoon red pepper flakes

INSTRUCTIONS:

1. In a large bowl, combine the romaine lettuce, spinach, bell pepper, cucumber, red onion, olives, feta cheese, and parsley.

2. In a separate bowl, whisk together the olive oil, red wine vinegar, honey, garlic powder, oregano, and red pepper flakes.

3. Pour the dressing over the salad and toss to combine.

4. Serve and enjoy!

4. Mediterranean Farro Salad

INGREDIENTS:

- 2 cups farro

- 4 cups vegetable broth

- 2 tablespoons olive oil

- 2 tablespoons lemon juice

- 1 teaspoon garlic powder

- 1/2 teaspoon oregano

- 1/4 teaspoon red pepper flakes

- 1/2 cup diced tomatoes

- 1/2 cup diced cucumber

- 1/2 cup kalamata olives, pitted and halved

- 1/4 cup feta cheese, crumbled

- 2 tablespoons fresh parsley, finely chopped

INSTRUCTIONS:

1. Bring the vegetable broth to a boil in a medium saucepan.

2. Stir in the farro and reduce heat to low.

3. Cover and cook for 15-20 minutes, or until the farro is tender.

4. Remove from heat and fluff with a fork.

5. In a small bowl, whisk together the olive oil, lemon juice, garlic powder, oregano, and red pepper flakes.

6. In a large bowl, combine the cooked farro, tomatoes, cucumber, olives, feta cheese, and parsley.

7. Pour the dressing over the salad and toss to combine.

8. Serve and enjoy!

5. Mediterranean Quinoa Salad

INGREDIENTS:

- 2 cups quinoa

- 4 cups vegetable broth

- 2 tablespoons olive oil

- 2 tablespoons lemon juice

- 1 teaspoon garlic powder

- 1/2 teaspoon oregano

- 1/4 teaspoon red pepper flakes

- 1/2 cup diced tomatoes

- 1/2 cup diced cucumber

- 1/2 cup kalamata olives, pitted and halved

- 1/4 cup feta cheese, crumbled

- 2 tablespoons fresh parsley, finely chopped

INSTRUCTIONS:

1. Bring the vegetable broth to a boil in a medium saucepan.

2. Stir in the quinoa and reduce heat to low.

3. Cover and cook for 15-20 minutes, or until the quinoa is tender.

4. Remove from heat and fluff with a fork.

5. In a small bowl, whisk together the olive oil, lemon juice, garlic powder, oregano, and red pepper flakes.

6. In a large bowl, combine the cooked quinoa, tomatoes, cucumber, olives, feta cheese, and parsley.

7. Pour the dressing over the salad and toss to combine.

8. Serve and enjoy!

6. Mediterranean Orzo Salad

INGREDIENTS:

- 2 cups orzo

- 4 cups vegetable broth

- 2 tablespoons olive oil

- 2 tablespoons lemon juice

- 1 teaspoon garlic powder

- 1/2 teaspoon oregano

- 1/4 teaspoon red pepper flakes

- 1/2 cup diced tomatoes

- 1/2 cup diced cucumber

- 1/2 cup kalamata olives, pitted and halved

- 1/4 cup feta cheese, crumbled

- 2 tablespoons fresh parsley, finely chopped

INSTRUCTIONS:

1. Bring the vegetable broth to a boil in a medium saucepan.

2. Stir in the orzo and reduce heat to low.

3. Cover and cook for 8-10 minutes, or until the orzo is tender.

4. Remove from heat and fluff with a fork.

5. In a small bowl, whisk together the olive oil, lemon juice, garlic powder, oregano, and red pepper flakes.

6. In a large bowl, combine the cooked orzo, tomatoes, cucumber, olives, feta cheese, and parsley.

7. Pour the dressing over the salad and toss to combine.

8. Serve and enjoy!

7. Mediterranean White Bean Salad

INGREDIENTS:

- 2 cans white beans, drained and rinsed

- 2 tablespoons olive oil

- 2 tablespoons lemon juice

- 1 teaspoon garlic powder

- 1/2 teaspoon oregano

- 1/4 teaspoon red pepper flakes

- 1/2 cup diced tomatoes

- 1/2 cup diced cucumber

- 1/2 cup kalamata olives, pitted and halved

- 1/4 cup feta cheese, crumbled

- 2 tablespoons fresh parsley, finely chopped

INSTRUCTIONS:

1. In a large bowl, combine the beans, tomatoes, cucumber, olives, feta cheese, and parsley.

2. In a small bowl, whisk together the olive oil, lemon juice, garlic powder, oregano, and red pepper flakes.

3. Pour the dressing over the salad and toss to combine.

4. Serve and enjoy!

8. Mediterranean Chickpea Salad

INGREDIENTS:

- 2 cans chickpeas, drained and rinsed

- 2 tablespoons olive oil

- 2 tablespoons lemon juice

- 1 teaspoon garlic powder

- 1/2 teaspoon oregano

- 1/4 teaspoon red pepper flakes

- 1/2 cup diced tomatoes

- 1/2 cup diced cucumber

- 1/2 cup kalamata olives, pitted and halved

- 1/4 cup feta cheese, crumbled

- 2 tablespoons fresh parsley, finely chopped

INSTRUCTIONS:

1. In a large bowl, combine the chickpeas, tomatoes, cucumber, olives, feta cheese, and parsley.

2. In a small bowl, whisk together the olive oil, lemon juice, garlic powder, oregano, and red pepper flakes.

3. Pour the dressing over the salad and toss to combine.

4. Serve and enjoy!

9. Mediterranean Lentil Salad

INGREDIENTS:

- 2 cups green lentils, cooked

- 2 tablespoons olive oil

- 2 tablespoons lemon juice

- 1 teaspoon garlic powder

- 1/2 teaspoon oregano

- 1/4 teaspoon red pepper flakes

- 1/2 cup diced tomatoes

- 1/2 cup diced cucumber

- 1/2 cup kalamata olives, pitted and halved

- 1/4 cup feta cheese, crumbled

- 2 tablespoons fresh parsley, finely chopped

INSTRUCTIONS:

1. In a large bowl, combine the cooked lentils, tomatoes, cucumber, olives, feta cheese, and parsley.

2. In a small bowl, whisk together the olive oil, lemon juice, garlic powder, oregano, and red pepper flakes.

3. Pour the dressing over the salad and toss to combine.

4. Serve and enjoy!

10. Mediterranean Feta Salad

INGREDIENTS:

- 2 cups baby spinach

- 1 cup diced tomatoes

- 1/2 cup diced cucumber

- 1/2 cup kalamata olives, pitted and halved

- 1/4 cup feta cheese, crumbled

- 2 tablespoons olive oil

- 2 tablespoons red wine vinegar

- 2 teaspoons honey

- 1/2 teaspoon garlic powder

- 1/4 teaspoon oregano

- 1/4 teaspoon red pepper flakes

INSTRUCTIONS:

1. In a large bowl, combine the spinach, tomatoes, cucumber, olives, and feta cheese.

2. In a small bowl, whisk together the olive oil, red wine vinegar, honey, garlic powder, oregano, and red pepper flakes.

3. Pour the dressing over the salad and toss to combine.

4. Serve and enjoy!

CHAPTER EIGHT

MEDITERRANEAN SNACKS AND APETIZERS

1. Hummus

INGREDIENTS:

- 1 can (15 ounces) of chickpeas, drained and rinsed

- 2 cloves garlic, minced

- 2 tablespoons of tahini

- 2 tablespoons of fresh lemon juice

- 2 tablespoons of olive oil

- 1/2 teaspoon of ground cumin

- Salt and pepper to taste

INSTRUCTIONS:

- Place all ingredients in a food processor and blend until smooth.

- Serve with pita bread, crackers, or vegetables.

2. Greek Yogurt Dip

INGREDIENTS:

- 1 cup plain Greek yogurt

- 2 tablespoons of olive oil

- 2 tablespoons of chopped fresh herbs (such as dill, parsley, or oregano)

- 2 cloves garlic, minced

- Salt and pepper to taste

INSTRUCTIONS:

- In a medium bowl, combine all ingredients and mix until well blended.

- Serve with pita bread, crackers, or vegetables.

3. Olive Tapenade

INGREDIENTS:

- 1 cup of black olives, pitted and chopped

- 2 cloves garlic, minced

- 2 tablespoons of capers

- 2 tablespoons of olive oil

- Juice of 1 lemon

- 1 teaspoon of fresh thyme

- Salt and pepper to taste

INSTRUCTIONS:

- Place all ingredients in a food processor and blend until smooth.

- Serve with pita bread, crackers, or vegetables.

4. Feta-Stuffed Mushrooms

INGREDIENTS:

- 10 large mushrooms, stems removed

- 1/2 cup crumbled feta cheese

- 2 tablespoons of olive oil

- 2 tablespoons of minced fresh parsley

- 1/4 teaspoon of ground cumin

- Salt and pepper to taste

INSTRUCTIONS:

- Preheat oven to 350 degrees F.

- In a medium bowl, combine feta cheese, olive oil, parsley, cumin, salt and pepper.

- Stuff each mushroom with the feta mixture.

- Place mushrooms on a baking sheet and bake for 20 minutes, or until mushrooms are tender.

5. Grilled Eggplant Dip

INGREDIENTS:

- 1 large eggplant

- 2 tablespoons of olive oil

- 2 cloves garlic, minced

- Juice of 1 lemon

- 2 tablespoons of tahini

- Salt and pepper to taste

INSTRUCTIONS:

- Preheat grill to medium-high heat.

- Slice eggplant in half lengthwise.

- Brush eggplant halves with olive oil and place on the grill. Grill for 10 minutes, or until eggplant is tender.

- Remove eggplant from the grill and let cool.

- Scoop out the flesh of the eggplant and place in a food processor.

- Add garlic, lemon juice, tahini, salt and pepper and blend until smooth.

- Serve with pita bread, crackers, or vegetables.

6. Baba Ganoush

INGREDIENTS:

- 1 large eggplant

- 2 cloves garlic, minced

- 2 tablespoons of tahini

- Juice of 1 lemon

- 2 tablespoons of olive oil

- Salt and pepper to taste

INSTRUCTIONS:

- Preheat oven to 375 degrees F.

- Pierce eggplant with a fork and place on a baking sheet.

- Bake for 40 minutes, or until eggplant is tender.

- Let eggplant cool, then scoop out the flesh.

- Place eggplant flesh in a food processor with garlic, tahini, lemon juice, olive oil, salt and pepper.

- Blend until smooth.

- Serve with pita bread, crackers, or vegetables.

7. Roasted Red Pepper Dip

INGREDIENTS:

- 2 red bell peppers

- 2 tablespoons of olive oil

- 2 cloves garlic, minced

- 2 tablespoons of tahini

- Juice of 1 lemon

- Salt and pepper to taste

INSTRUCTIONS:

- Preheat oven to 400 degrees F.

- Place red bell peppers on a baking sheet and roast for 30 minutes, or until peppers are tender and skins are blackened.

- Let peppers cool and remove the skins.

- Place peppers in a food processor with garlic, tahini, lemon juice, olive oil, salt and pepper.

- Blend until smooth.

- Serve with pita bread, crackers, or vegetables.

8. Grilled Zucchini Rounds

INGREDIENTS:

- 2 zucchini, sliced into 1/4 inch rounds

- 2 tablespoons of olive oil

- Juice of 1 lemon

- 1 teaspoon of fresh oregano

- Salt and pepper to taste

INSTRUCTIONS:

- Preheat grill to medium-high heat.

- Brush zucchini rounds with olive oil and place on the grill. Grill for 4 minutes per side, or until lightly charred and tender.

- Place grilled zucchini rounds on a platter and top with lemon juice, oregano, salt and pepper.

- Serve with pita bread, crackers, or vegetables.

9. Greek Salad Skewers

INGREDIENTS:

- 1 cucumber, cut into 1-inch cubes

- 1/2 red onion, cut into 1-inch cubes

- 1/2 cup cherry tomatoes

- 1/2 cup kalamata olives

- 1/2 cup feta cheese, crumbled

- 2 tablespoons of olive oil

- Juice of 1 lemon

- 2 tablespoons of fresh oregano

- Salt and pepper to taste

INSTRUCTIONS:

- Preheat grill to medium-high heat.

- Using metal or wooden skewers, thread cucumber cubes, red onion cubes, cherry tomatoes, olives, and feta cheese onto each skewer.

- Brush skewers with olive oil and place on the grill. Grill for 5 minutes per side, or until lightly charred and vegetables are tender.

- Place skewers on a platter and top with lemon juice, oregano, salt and pepper.

- Serve with pita bread, crackers, or vegetables.

10. Falafel

INGREDIENTS:

- 1 can (15 ounces) of chickpeas, drained and rinsed

- 2 cloves garlic, minced

- 1/2 cup fresh parsley, chopped

- 1/2 cup fresh cilantro, chopped

- 2 tablespoons of ground cumin

- 2 tablespoons of olive oil

- 2 tablespoons of flour

- Salt and pepper to taste

INSTRUCTIONS:

- Place all ingredients in a food processor and blend until smooth.

- Form into 1-inch balls and place on a baking sheet.

- Preheat oven to 350 degrees F.

- Bake falafel for 20 minutes, or until lightly golden.

- Serve with pita bread, crackers, or vegetables.

CHAPTER NINE

TIPS FOR EATING A MEDITERRANEAN DIET

1. Start with the basics: The cornerstone of the Mediterranean diet is fruits, vegetables, whole grains, legumes, and nuts. Fill half your plate with colorful vegetables and fruits, and choose whole grains like barley, quinoa, and oats.

2. Increase your healthy fats: The Mediterranean diet is known for its emphasis on healthy fats. Reach for foods like extra-virgin olive oil, avocados, nuts, and seeds to boost your healthy fat intake.

3. Use herbs and spices: Herbs and spices are a great way to boost flavor without adding extra calories or fat. Try adding oregano, basil, rosemary, garlic, or cinnamon to your dishes for a flavor boost.

4. Eat seafood: Seafood is a great source of lean protein and omega-3 fatty acids. Aim to consume fish at least twice a week.

5. Take pleasure in your meals: Eating should be a fun experience. Take time to savor your food and enjoy the company of others.

6. Limit processed and refined foods: Processed and refined foods are high in unhealthy fats and calories and have no nutritional value. Avoid processed meats, such as bacon and sausage, as well as processed snacks, such as chips and candy.

8. Exercise regularly and stay hydrated: Exercise is an important part of a healthy lifestyle. Every week, aim for at least 150 minutes of moderate-intensity exercise. Keep your body hydrated by drinking plenty of water throughout the day.

PREPARING MEALS

Preparing meals for a Mediterranean diet is both delicious and nutritious. The Mediterranean diet is based on the traditional eating habits of people living in Greece, Spain, and other countries that border the Mediterranean Sea. This diet is high in fresh fruits, vegetables, whole grains, beans, nuts, and olive oil. Seafood, poultry, and eggs are also a part of the Mediterranean diet.

1. Start with fresh ingredients. When preparing a Mediterranean meal, it is best to use fresh ingredients whenever possible. Choose seasonal fruits and vegetables and local, sustainable sources of seafood and poultry.

2. Add healthy fats. Olive oil is a staple ingredient in Mediterranean cooking and provides a good source of healthy fats. You can also add nuts, such as walnuts, almonds, and pine nuts, to salads or dishes to add flavor and nutrition.

3. Get creative with herbs and spices. Add herbs and spices to your meals to make them tastier. Popular Mediterranean herbs and spices include oregano, thyme, basil, parsley, garlic, and pepper.

4. Use whole grains. Whole grains such as quinoa, bulgur, and farro are an important part of the Mediterranean diet. Use them in place of refined grains like white rice or pasta.

5. Make your meals colorful. To create a visually appealing meal, include a variety of colors in your dishes. Fruits and vegetables such as tomatoes, bell peppers, eggplant, and mushrooms add bright hues and nutrition to your plate.

Following the Mediterranean diet can help you maintain a healthy lifestyle. By preparing meals with fresh ingredients, healthy fats, herbs, spices, and whole grains, you can create delicious and nutritious Mediterranean-style meals.

CONCLUSION

The Mediterranean Diet Cookbook is an ideal resource for anyone looking to explore the flavors and recipes of the Mediterranean Diet. With an array of recipes for all courses, from breakfast to dessert, this cookbook offers something for everyone. The recipes are all easy to follow and don't require any specialized cooking skills or ingredients. They are all healthy, delicious, and will help you get the most out of the Mediterranean Diet. With this cookbook, you can enjoy the fresh flavors and health benefits of the Mediterranean Diet without having to travel to the Mediterranean. Enjoy the flavors of the Mediterranean in your own kitchen!